Greenwillow
Read-alone

JUDITH S. SEIXAS

DRUGS
WHAT THEY ARE,
WHAT THEY DO

illustrated by TOM HUFFMAN

GREENWILLOW BOOKS, New York

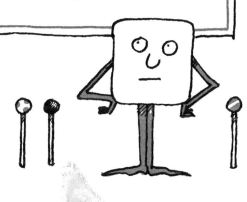

This book is dedicated to Susan Hirschman
who has guided me, gently but firmly,
into the world of writing. —J.S.S.

With love for Adam J. —T.H.

Library of Congress Cataloging-in-Publication
Seixas, Judith S.
Drugs—what they are, what they do.
(Greenwillow read-alone books)
Summary: An easy-to-read guide to
psychoactive drugs and how they change
the way we feel, think, and act.
1. Psychotropic drugs—Juvenile literature.
2. Substance abuse—Juvenile literature.
[1. Psychotropic drugs. 2. Drug abuse]
I. Huffman, Tom. ill. II. Title. III. Series.
RM315.S45 1987 616.86'3 86-336
ISBN 0-688-07399-9
ISBN 0-688-07400-6 (lib. bdg.)

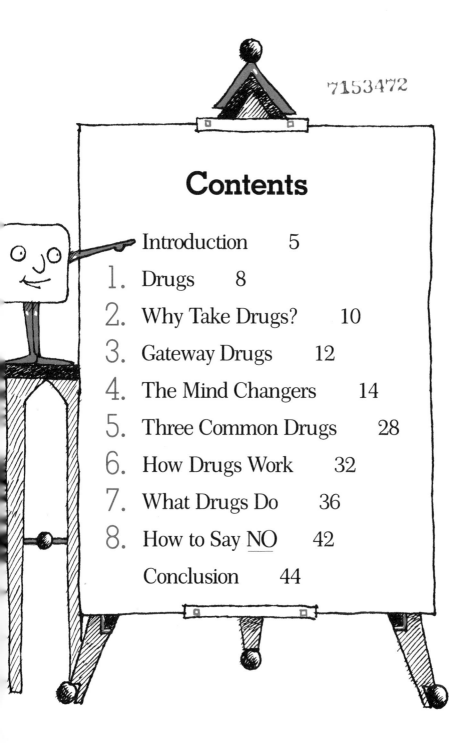

Contents

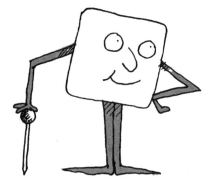

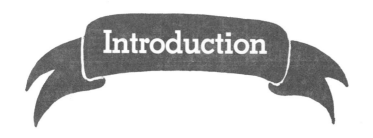

Introduction

A drug is any chemical
that changes the way
our minds and bodies work.
Aspirin, tea, penicillin,
and alcohol are all drugs.

THIS BOOK IS ABOUT
PSYCHOACTIVE DRUGS ONLY.

Psychoactive drugs change
how we feel, think, and act.

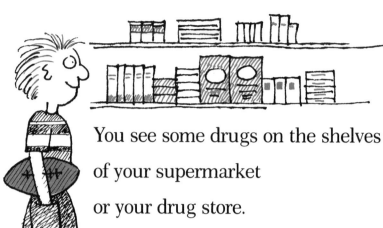

You see some drugs on the shelves

of your supermarket

or your drug store.

Some may be given to you

for a sore throat or a fever.

Others may be ordered by a doctor.

A doctor will tell you

exactly how much of a drug

to use so that it will be safe.

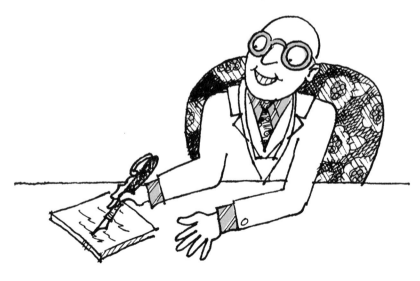

Most psychoactive drugs
are illegal.
They cannot be given
to you by anyone,
even a parent or a doctor.
It is against the law
for you to buy, sell,
or use them.

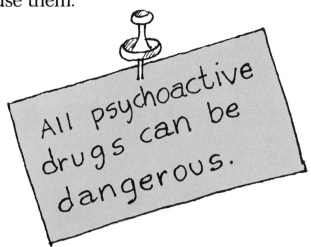

All psychoactive
drugs can be
dangerous.

1. Drugs

Drugs are not new.
They have been used
for thousands of years
to kill pain or cure sickness.
At least 700 different drugs
were used by ancient Greeks,
Egyptians, and Arabs.
They were thought to have
the power of magic.

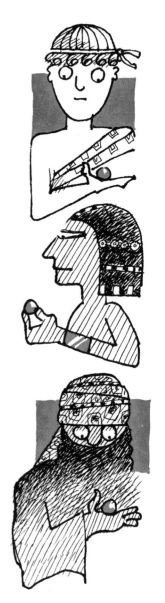

8

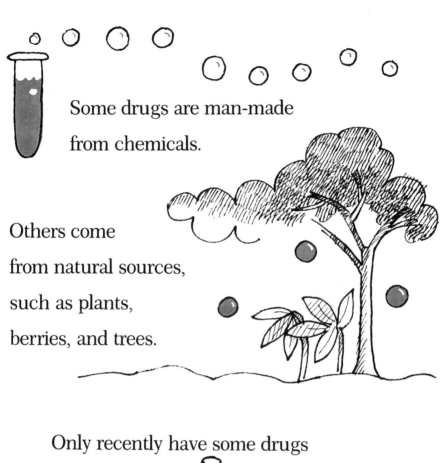

Some drugs are man-made from chemicals.

Others come from natural sources, such as plants, berries, and trees.

Only recently have some drugs become illegal.

They are illegal because we now know how much harm they can do.

2. Why Take Drugs?

If drugs are so harmful,
why do young people try them?
Here are some reasons
they give:

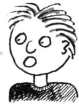

to have fun and
fit in with friends,

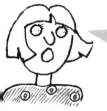

out of curiosity to see
how drugs make them feel,

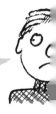

because they were told drugs
make you forget about bad feelings,

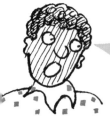

because a friend dared them
to try something new,

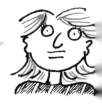

because they didn't know
how to say NO.

All these reasons

do not change

what drugs will do.

Young people do not talk

about the bad effects.

They think nothing

can harm them.

They think that people

try to scare them

by making drugs

sound worse than they are.

BUT THIS IS NOT SO.

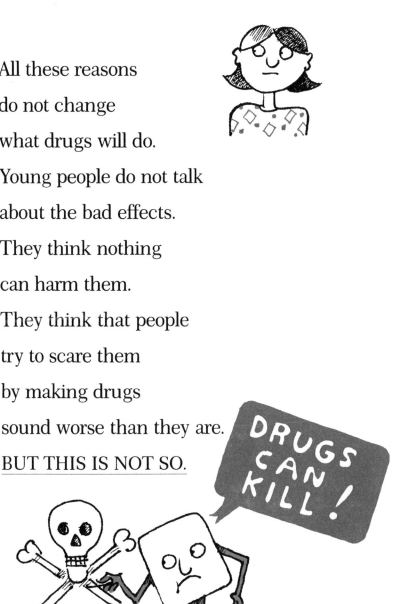

3. Gateway Drugs

The drugs you may be
tempted by first
are called *"gateway drugs."*
They are TOBACCO, ALCOHOL,
and MARIJUANA.
You may have already
used one of them.
You may have tried a puff
on a cigarette.
Or you may have had
a sip of beer.
You may have heard,
"Try it once, it's fun."

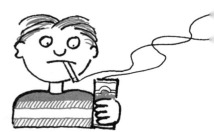

Young people who use
tobacco and alcohol
are more likely
to try marijuana.
Then they may go on
to stronger drugs.
Researchers have found:

If you do not use
"gateway" drugs,
there is a better chance
that you will never use
other harmful drugs.

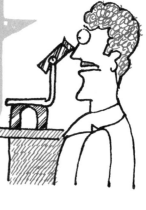

4. The Mind Changers

Stimulants, sedatives, hallucinogens, and narcotics are all psychoactive drugs.

STIMULANTS

Stimulants are called "uppers," "pep pills," or "speed." They make you feel restless. People take stimulants to keep awake.

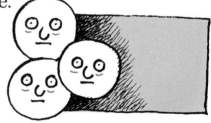

Some students

take them before a test,

so they can stay up all night to study.

These drugs raise blood pressure.

They strain the heart.

They can even cause heart attacks.

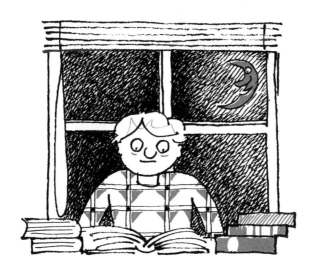

COCAINE "(coke)"

is the most widely used

illegal stimulant.

It is a white powder

made from coca leaves.

Cocaine is usually

sniffed or snorted.

It raises blood pressure

and can numb

parts of the body.

When it is sniffed daily,

cocaine will cause

painful sores

and

a runny nose.

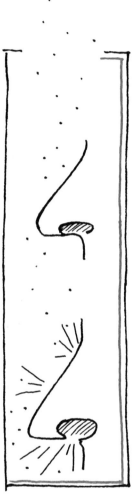

If the user keeps on snorting,

the drug will make a hole

from nostril to nostril.

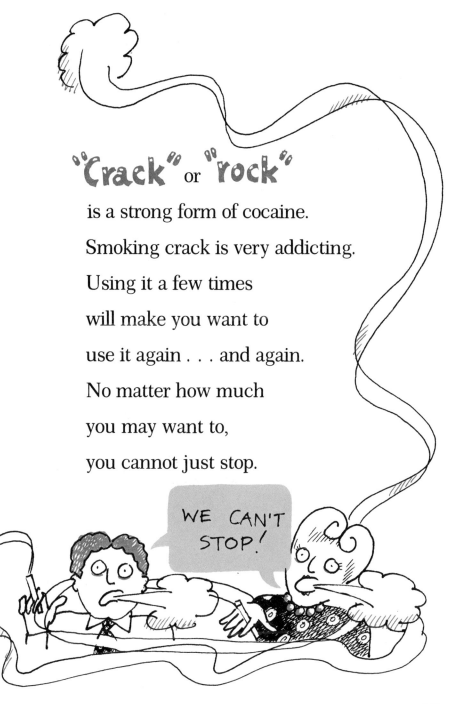

"Crack" or "rock"

is a strong form of cocaine.

Smoking crack is very addicting.

Using it a few times

will make you want to

use it again . . . and again.

No matter how much

you may want to,

you cannot just stop.

WE CAN'T STOP!

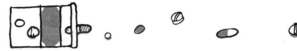

SEDATIVES

Sedatives are called **"downers."**

They calm you.

Sedatives include all sleeping pills

and tranquilizers.

If they are not ordered by a doctor,

they are illegal.

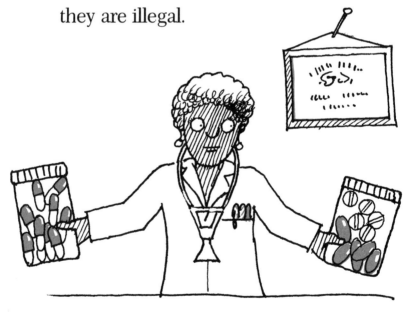

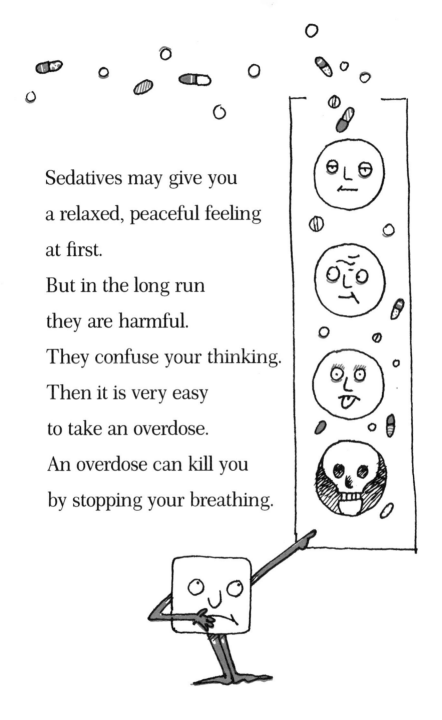

Sedatives may give you
a relaxed, peaceful feeling
at first.
But in the long run
they are harmful.
They confuse your thinking.
Then it is very easy
to take an overdose.
An overdose can kill you
by stopping your breathing.

HALLUCINOGENS

Hallucinogens distort reality.

They distort how you hear,

feel, and see.

A scratch on a desk

may look like

a wriggling snake.

Hallucinogens include:

- LSD, which is known as "acid"
- PCP, which is often called "angel dust"
- INHALANTS
- MARIJUANA

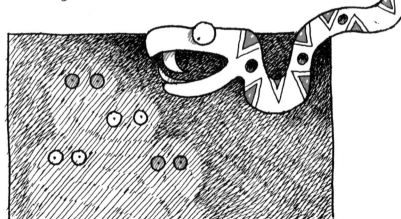

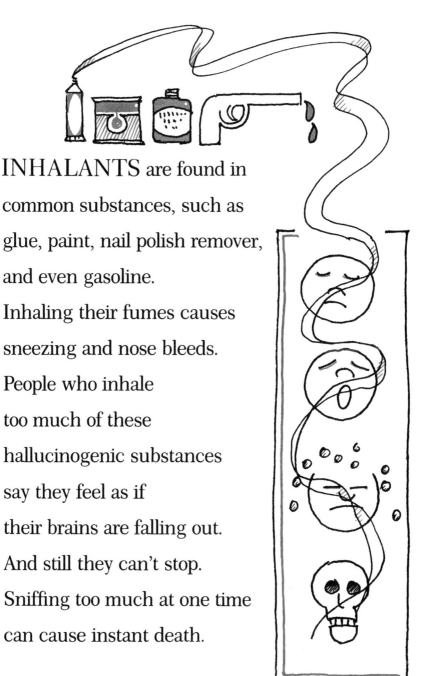

INHALANTS are found in
common substances, such as
glue, paint, nail polish remover,
and even gasoline.
Inhaling their fumes causes
sneezing and nose bleeds.
People who inhale
too much of these
hallucinogenic substances
say they feel as if
their brains are falling out.
And still they can't stop.
Sniffing too much at one time
can cause instant death.

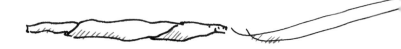

MARIJUANA

is a mild hallucinogen,

but it is the one

that is most widely used.

It is known as

"grass" or "pot".

It is smoked in

"reefers" or "joints"

that look like small cigarettes.

Marijuana can also be eaten.

Hashish ("hash")

is a strong form

of marijuana.

Until recently,
scientists thought that
marijuana was not harmful.
But research has shown
that this is not the case.

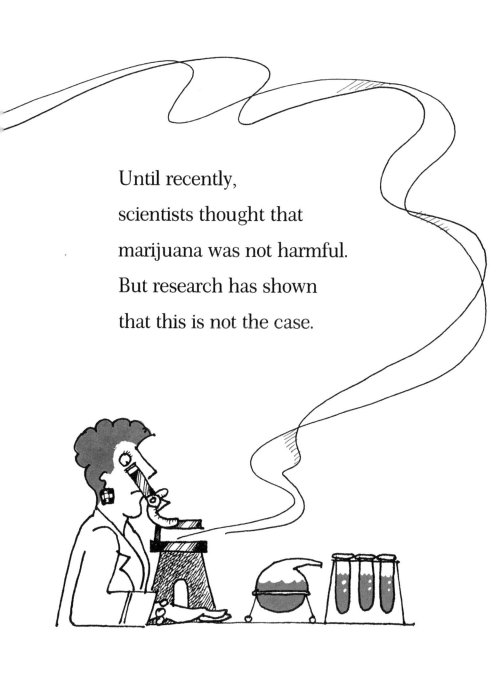

NARCOTICS

Narcotics are used to calm you,

to lessen pain,

or to bring on sleep.

Narcotics include:

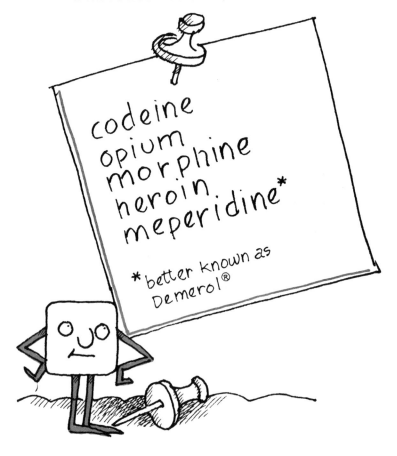

codeine
opium
morphine
heroin
meperidine*

* better known as
Demerol®

Narcotics blot out the real world.

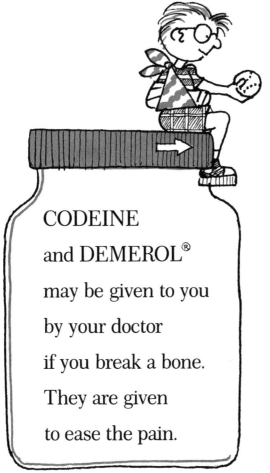

CODEINE

and DEMEROL®

may be given to you

by your doctor

if you break a bone.

They are given

to ease the pain.

They should never be used,

except for medical reasons.

HEROIN

is the most commonly used
illegal narcotic.
It has no known medical use.
Heroin gives users
a feeling of well-being
for a short time.
But it is soon followed by
sickness and depression.
Heroin also causes cramps,
watery eyes, clammy skin,
and nausea.

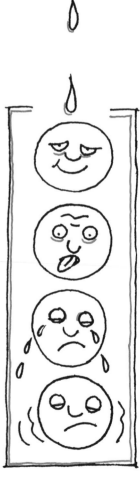

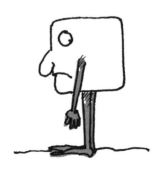

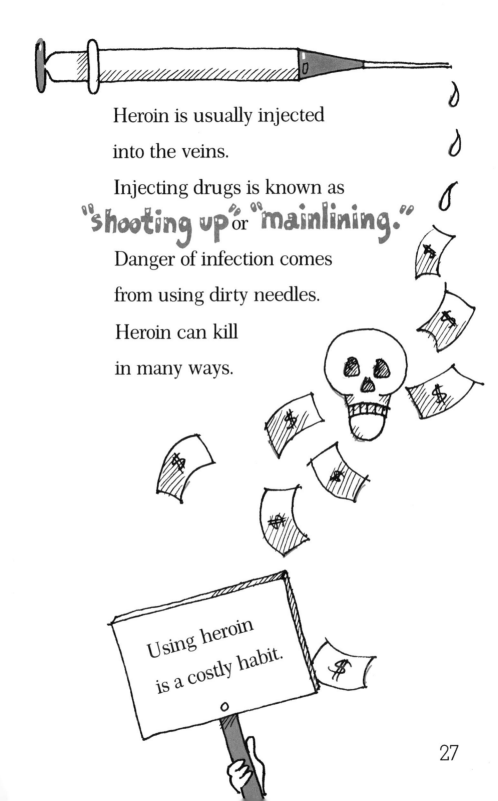

Heroin is usually injected
into the veins.
Injecting drugs is known as
"shooting up" or "mainlining."
Danger of infection comes
from using dirty needles.
Heroin can kill
in many ways.

Using heroin
is a costly habit.

27

5. Three Common Drugs

There are three drugs
that affect our moods
and mental state.
Because they are so commonly used,
we don't realize what they can do.
They are:

- CAFFEINE, found in tea, coffee,
  cocoa, and cola drinks,
- NICOTINE, found in tobaccos,
- ALCOHOL, found in beer, wine,
  and hard liquor.

Even though caffeine, nicotine,
and alcohol are legal drugs,
they are dangerous.

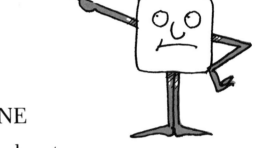

CAFFEINE

strains the heart.
Too much caffeine
can make you jittery.

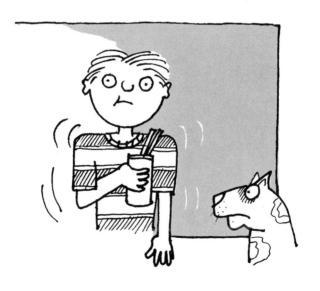

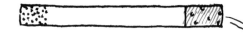

NICOTINE, which is smoked in tobacco,

is also a strain on the heart.

In addition to nicotine, tobacco

contains other chemicals.

When these chemicals are inhaled,

they cause many diseases.

Lung cancer is one of them.

Yet people smoke even after

they read the label

on cigarette packages,

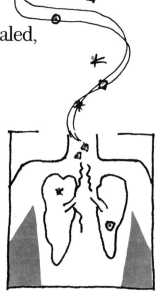

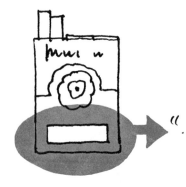

"...cigarette smoking is
dangerous to your health

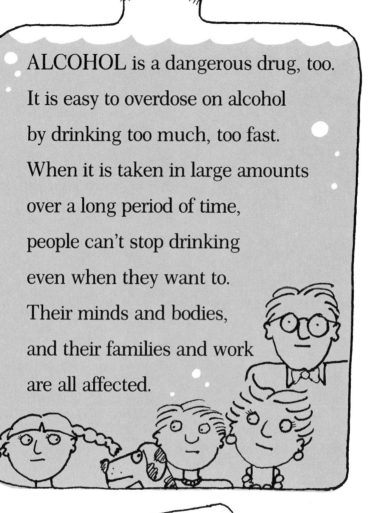

ALCOHOL is a dangerous drug, too. It is easy to overdose on alcohol by drinking too much, too fast. When it is taken in large amounts over a long period of time, people can't stop drinking even when they want to. Their minds and bodies, and their families and work are all affected.

In most states you must be twenty-one years old to buy alcohol.

31

6. How Drugs Work

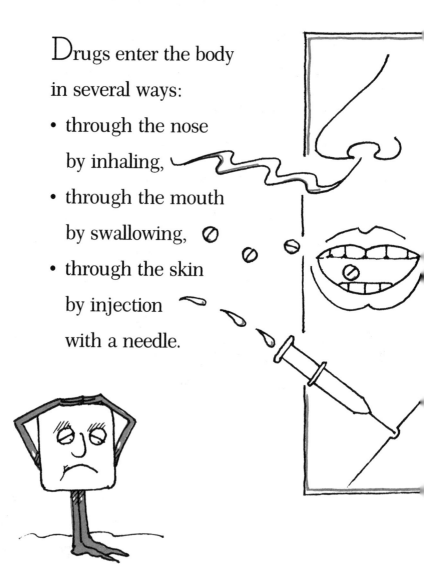

Drugs enter the body
in several ways:
- through the nose
  by inhaling,
- through the mouth
  by swallowing,
- through the skin
  by injection
  with a needle.

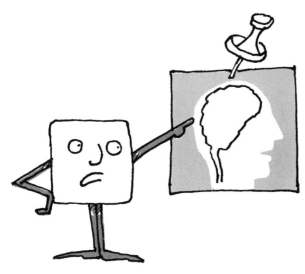

No matter how a drug

gets into your body,

it goes to your brain.

It gets there by way

of the bloodstream.

Drugs affect

different people

in different ways.

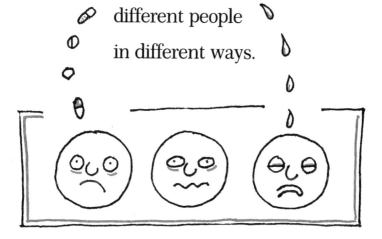

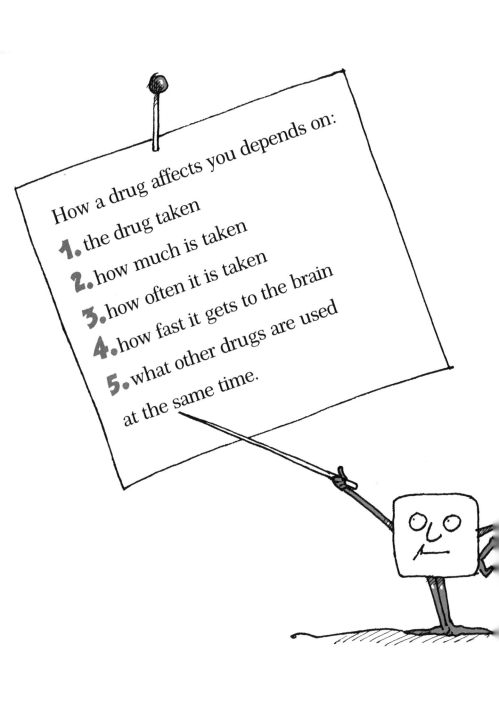

How a drug affects you depends on:

1. the drug taken
2. how much is taken
3. how often it is taken
4. how fast it gets to the brain
5. what other drugs are used at the same time.

Some drugs get to the brain
in a few seconds.
Others take much longer.
The effects of some drugs
last for hours, days,
weeks, or years.

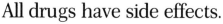

All drugs have side effects.
For example, people who
drink too much alcohol
may feel cheered up
at first.
Later they get sick,
or have a terrible
hangover.

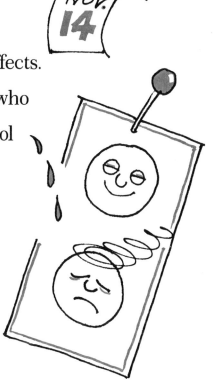

7. What Drugs Do

PSYCHOACTIVE DRUGS

If you take
a psychoactive drug,
you may feel
sleepy or dizzy.
Most of these drugs
make you feel good
at first, but
soon they will make
you feel sick or sad.
Psychoactive drugs
make you think
you can do things
you really cannot do.

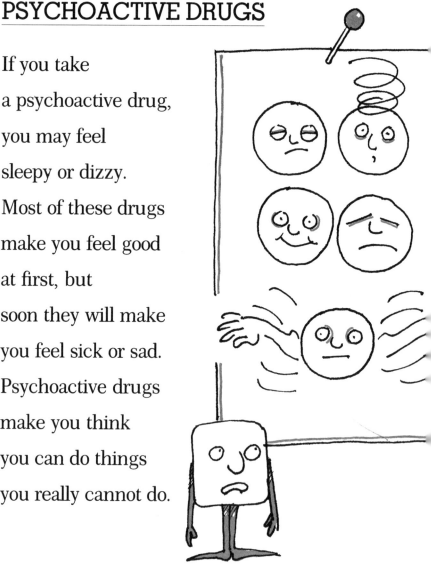

36

ADDICTION

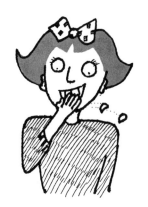

Do you bite
your fingernails?
If you do,
you probably hate
how your nails look.
A parent may have told you
to stop biting them.
You may have
tried hard to stop.
But you couldn't.

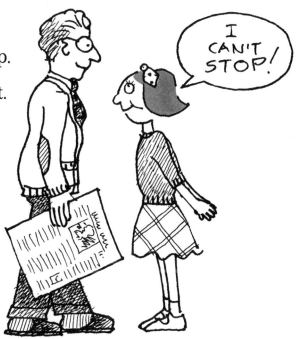

I CAN'T STOP!

As hard as this was,

it is much harder

for an addict

to stop using drugs,

no matter how much

he wants to.

He needs the drug to feel normal.

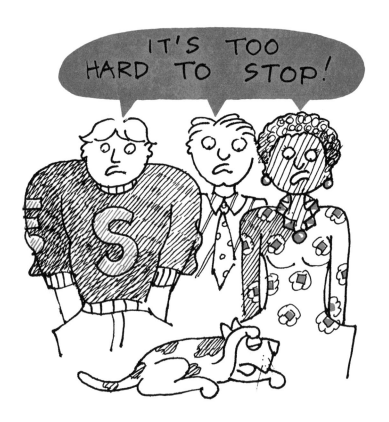

Often people who were honest
and hard-working
before they took drugs
become drug addicts.
Then they lie, steal,
and cheat to pay for
the drugs they need.

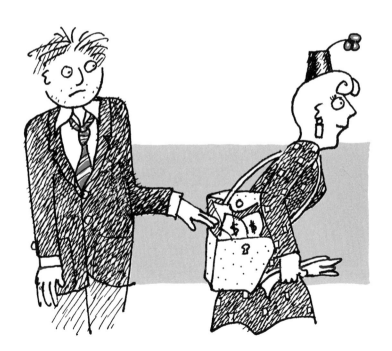

TOLERANCE

When people take a drug

for a long time,

they develop a tolerance for it.

Their bodies need

more and more of the drug

to get the same effect.

It is like jumping

into cold water.

At first you feel very cold.

But soon your body

gets used to it.

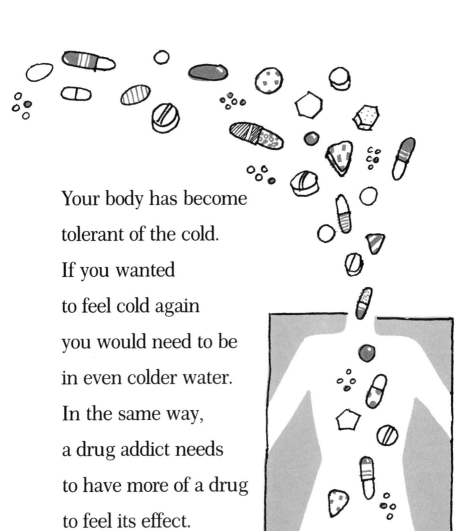

Your body has become
tolerant of the cold.
If you wanted
to feel cold again
you would need to be
in even colder water.
In the same way,
a drug addict needs
to have more of a drug
to feel its effect.

8. How to Say NO

At some time
friends will urge you
to try drugs.
They are not real friends.
Real friends help friends say NO.

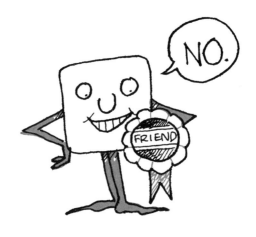

If you are tempted
you can say:

- NO.

- No, thank you!

- No, I'm not into drugs.

- No, I have other things to do:

I'm playing ball today.

I'm riding my bike.

Dad and I are going shopping.

I have a good book to read.

- Or,

JUST SAY NO.

Ask your friends
to say NO, too.

Conclusion

You now know more
about what drugs do
to the mind and body.
You know why
they are harmful.

You understand
the troubles that come
from drug use.
You now know how easy it is
to become an addict.

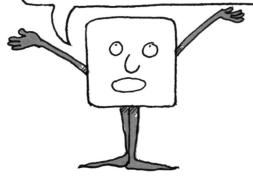

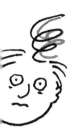

Any psychoactive drug will make it
difficult for you
to play catch or kick a ball.
You will be too dizzy to run.

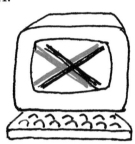

You will not be good
at computer games.

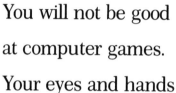

Your eyes and hands
will not work together.
The TV screen will look blurry.
You will be too mixed-up
to do school work
or learn anything.
You won't be able
to keep up with your friends.
They will wonder
what is wrong.

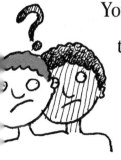

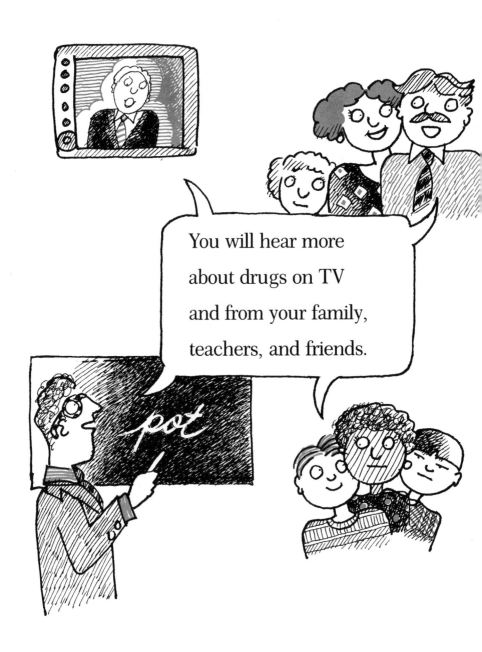

You will hear more about drugs on TV and from your family, teachers, and friends.

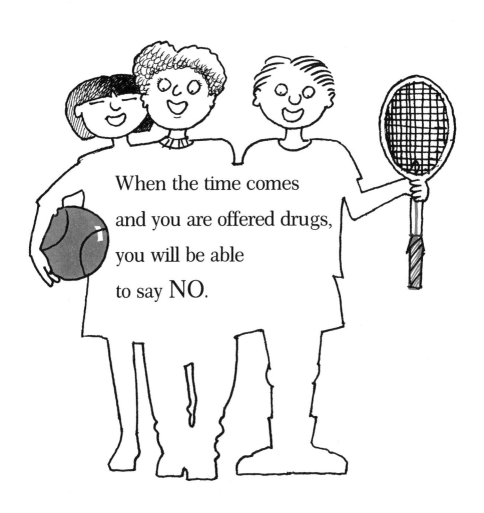

When the time comes
and you are offered drugs,
you will be able
to say NO.

JUDITH S. SEIXAS was graduated from Carleton College and has an M.A. from Columbia's Teachers College. She has long been involved in health issues, specializing in the treatment of alcoholics and their families. Her wide experience encompasses both the educational and the therapeutic. She is the co-author of *Children of Alcoholism: A Survivor's Manual* and for children the author of: *Water—What It Is, What It Does; Vitamins—What They Are, What They Do; Junk Food—What It Is, What It Does; Alcohol—What It Is, What It Does; Tobacco—What It Is, What It Does;* and *Living with a Parent Who Drinks Too Much.*

TOM HUFFMAN attended the School of Visual Arts in New York City and holds a B.A. from the University of Kentucky. Mr. Huffman is a free-lance artist whose works have appeared in galleries, advertisements, and national magazines. He has illustrated many children's books, including eight Greenwillow Read-alone Books.

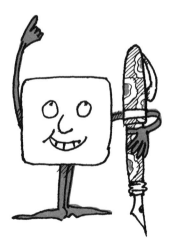